BLACK SEED OIL FOR SKIN TREATMENT

Unveiling Nature's Secret Elixir for Radiant Health and Timeless Beauty

Dr. Precious Eman

Contents

Introduction

In the ever-evolving landscape of skincare, where trends come and go like fleeting seasons, there exists a timeless elixir that has transcended centuries — Black Seed Oil. Nestled within the seeds of Nigella Sativa, this ancient remedy has resurfaced in the modern world, captivating skincare enthusiasts and health seekers alike with its remarkable benefits.

As we navigate a sea of beauty products promising miracles and magic, it's essential to return to the roots of holistic and natural healing. Black Seed Oil, celebrated for its multifaceted properties, emerges as a beacon of simplicity in a world often clouded by complex formulations and chemical concoctions.

This journey through the pages of "Black Seed Oil for Skin Treatment" is an exploration of the rich tapestry that is black seed oil. We will delve into the scientific intricacies of its composition, unravel the historical threads that have woven its story through time, and most importantly, discover how this humble oil can revolutionize your skincare routine.

This book is not just a guide; it's an invitation to rediscover the age-old wisdom that our ancestors held dear. As we traverse the realms of acne, aging, and other common skin woes, black seed oil will emerge as a steadfast companion, offering a natural and holistic approach to nurturing your skin.

Through this book, you will witness the alchemy of black seed oil unfold — from its potent anti-inflammatory effects to its role in combating the signs of aging. We will share practical tips on incorporating black seed oil seamlessly into your daily skincare rituals, backed by personal testimonials and expert insights.

Beyond the mirror's reflection lies a deeper connection between inner well-being and outer radiance. "Black Seed Oil for Skin Treatment" is not just about treating the skin; it's about celebrating the beauty that arises when we care for ourselves holistically.

Join us on this voyage of self-discovery, as we unlock the secrets of black seed oil, a gift from nature that promises not just a radiant complexion but a holistic embrace of well-being. Your journey to luminous and healthy skin begins here.

Definition and Origins of Black Seed Oil (Nigella Sativa)

Definition:

Black seed oil, derived from the seeds of Nigella Sativa, is a versatile and potent natural remedy known for its therapeutic properties. Also referred to as black cumin seed oil or kalonji oil, it has been utilized for centuries in traditional medicine systems across various cultures for its remarkable health and skincare benefits.

The oil itself is extracted through a cold-pressing method, preserving its rich nutritional profile. Composed of a complex array of active compounds, black seed oil is characterized by its distinct aromatic flavor and is often employed both internally and externally for its diverse healing capabilities.

Origins:

Nigella Sativa, the plant from which black seed oil originates, is native to the Mediterranean region, as well as parts of Asia and the Middle East. Historically, its use dates back to ancient Egypt, where it was reportedly found in the tomb of Tutankhamun, emphasizing its cultural and medicinal significance.

The plant thrives in climates with well-drained soil and is recognized for its delicate pale blue or white flowers. The seeds, encapsulated within the fruit of the plant, are small, black, and teardrop-shaped, hence the name "black seed." The extraction of oil from these seeds has been a cherished practice for generations, passed down through cultural traditions and wisdom.

Black seed oil's journey has transcended borders, finding its place in Ayurveda, Traditional Chinese

Medicine, and Islamic medicine, among other healing traditions. Today, its popularity has surged globally, as modern research continues to unveil its therapeutic potential and validate the wisdom embedded in its ancient origins.

Historical Uses and Cultural Significance of Black Seed Oil (Nigella Sativa)

In the Tapestry of Ancient Healing:

Black seed oil, with its origins deeply embedded in antiquity, has woven a rich tapestry of historical uses and cultural significance across diverse civilizations. Revered for its medicinal properties, this precious elixir has stood the test of time as a symbol of health and well-being.

Ancient Egypt: In the annals of history, black seed oil finds mention in the ancient civilization of Egypt, where it was reportedly discovered in the tomb of the iconic pharaoh Tutankhamun. Egyptians held the belief that the oil possessed transformative properties, emphasizing its inclusion among the treasures intended for the afterlife.

Ayurveda and Traditional Chinese Medicine: The influence of black seed oil extends far beyond the Nile. In Ayurveda, the traditional system of medicine in India, and Traditional Chinese Medicine, it has been embraced for its versatility. Both systems recognize its ability to balance the body and support overall health.

Islamic Tradition: Black seed oil occupies a special place in Islamic medicine and is mentioned in the hadith, the sayings of Prophet Muhammad. The Prophet himself reportedly declared, "In the black seed, there is a cure for every disease except death."

This proclamation has contributed to the widespread use of black seed oil in various Islamic cultures for a myriad of health concerns.

Mediterranean Folklore: Along the shores of the Mediterranean, where Nigella Sativa thrives, black seed oil has been integrated into traditional folk remedies. Its usage spans from promoting digestive health to addressing skin issues, reflecting a deep cultural connection to the bounties of the land.

Modern Resurgence: While rooted in ancient wisdom, black seed oil has experienced a modern resurgence, capturing the attention of a global audience. As scientific research continues to unveil its therapeutic potential, the cultural significance of black seed oil persists, serving as a bridge between ancient traditions and contemporary wellness practices.

Today, whether in the bustling markets of Marrakech, the spice bazaars of Istanbul, or the apothecaries of traditional healers, black seed oil stands as a testament to the enduring legacy of natural remedies and the interwoven threads of history and health.

Recent Resurgence in Popularity for Black Seed Oil in Skincare

In the ever-evolving landscape of skincare, where trends emerge and fade like seasons, there has been a notable and remarkable resurgence of interest in an ancient elixir – black seed oil. The recent years have witnessed a dynamic shift in consumer preferences towards natural and holistic approaches to skincare, catapulting black seed oil into the spotlight as a revered and sought-after ingredient.

1. Natural Skincare Movement: The resurgence of black seed oil aligns seamlessly with the broader natural skincare movement. Consumers are increasingly drawn to botanical solutions with a rich historical and cultural backdrop, seeking alternatives to synthetic and chemical-laden products. Black seed oil, with its time-tested efficacy, has become a beacon for those desiring a return to simplicity and authenticity in their skincare routines.

2. Scientific Validation: Advancements in scientific research have played a pivotal role in propelling black seed oil back into the limelight. Studies exploring its chemical composition and therapeutic properties have provided a solid foundation for the oil's credibility in skincare. The anti-inflammatory, antioxidant, and antimicrobial attributes of black seed oil, validated by modern science, have contributed to its popularity among those seeking evidence-backed solutions for common skin concerns.

3. Social Media Influence: The digital age has significantly contributed to the resurgence of black seed oil, with social media platforms serving as powerful catalysts for trends. Influencers, beauty enthusiasts, and skincare experts have shared their positive experiences with black seed oil, creating a ripple effect that has resonated with a global audience. The visual appeal of before-and-after transformations and the allure of natural remedies have propelled black seed oil into the skincare spotlight.

4. Conscious Consumerism: A growing awareness of sustainability and ethical sourcing has led consumers to seek products with a transparent and ethical supply chain. Black seed oil, often harvested from sustainable and organic sources, aligns with the values of conscious consumerism. This ethical dimension has further fueled its resurgence, making it a preferred choice for those mindful of the environmental and social impact of their skincare choices.

5. Holistic Wellness Approach: The integration of skincare into broader wellness practices has become a prevailing trend. Black seed oil, recognized not only for its topical benefits but also for its potential internal uses, resonates with individuals seeking a holistic approach to health. The idea of nurturing the skin from within has contributed to black seed oil's popularity as part of a comprehensive wellness strategy.

As we witness this resurgence, black seed oil stands as a testament to the enduring appeal of natural remedies in the dynamic world of skincare, proving that ancient wisdom can find a harmonious place in contemporary self-care rituals.

The Science behind Black Seed Oil: Nature's Healing Arsenal

1. Chemical Composition:

- **Thymoquinone:** The star player in black seed oil, thymoquinone is a powerful bioactive compound known for its anti-inflammatory and antioxidant properties. It has been the focus of numerous studies exploring its potential in combating various skin issues.

- **Fatty Acids:** Black seed oil boasts a rich profile of omega-3 and omega-6 fatty acids, crucial for maintaining skin health. These fatty acids contribute to the oil's moisturizing and nourishing qualities, promoting a supple and hydrated complexion.

- **Antioxidants:** Packed with antioxidants, black seed oil helps neutralize free radicals, preventing oxidative stress and the premature aging of the skin. This plays a vital role in maintaining skin elasticity and radiance.

2. *Anti-Inflammatory Properties:*

- Black seed oil is a potent anti-inflammatory agent, inhibiting pathways that lead to skin redness and swelling. This makes it particularly beneficial for those dealing with inflammatory skin conditions such as acne and eczema.

3. Antimicrobial Effects:

- The oil demonstrates antimicrobial activity against various pathogens, making it effective in addressing microbial imbalances on the skin. This property contributes to its use in treating acne and other skin blemishes.

4. Moisturizing and Nourishing Qualities:

- The combination of fatty acids and other nutrients in black seed oil makes it an excellent natural moisturizer. It helps lock in hydration, preventing dryness and flakiness. Additionally, the oil's nourishing properties contribute to overall skin health, supporting its natural barrier function.

5. Collagen Production and Anti-Aging:

- Black seed oil has been associated with the stimulation of collagen production, a crucial protein for maintaining skin firmness and elasticity. By promoting collagen synthesis, the oil contributes to reducing the appearance of fine lines and wrinkles.

6. Regulation of Sebum Production:

- For those grappling with oily or acne-prone skin, black seed oil offers a balancing act. It helps regulate sebum production, preventing excess oiliness and minimizing the risk of clogged pores that can lead to acne breakouts.

7. Free Radical Defense:

- The antioxidants present in black seed oil act as defenders against free radicals, which are molecules that can damage skin cells. This protective role helps in preventing premature aging and maintaining a youthful complexion.

Understanding the intricate science behind black seed oil sheds light on its multifaceted benefits for the skin. As we delve deeper into its chemical composition and mechanisms of action, the true potential of this natural elixir as a skincare ally becomes increasingly apparent.

Black Seed Oil and Common Skin Issues: A Natural Remedy Unveiled

1. Acne and Blemishes:

- **Reduction of Inflammation:** The anti-inflammatory properties of black seed oil make it a valuable asset in combating acne. By reducing inflammation, it helps soothe redness and discomfort associated with breakouts.

- **Control of Sebum Production:** Black seed oil aids in balancing sebum production, preventing excessive oiliness that can clog pores and contribute to acne development. This dual-action approach addresses both the symptoms and underlying causes of acne.

2. Eczema and Psoriasis:

- **Calming Irritated Skin:** Individuals dealing with eczema and psoriasis often experience irritated and inflamed skin. Black seed oil's anti-inflammatory compounds can provide relief, calming the skin and reducing the redness associated with these conditions.

- **Alleviating Itching and Redness:** The soothing properties of black seed oil extend to relieving itching and discomfort, offering a natural alternative for those seeking relief from the symptoms of eczema and psoriasis.

3. Aging and Wrinkles:

- **Antioxidant Protection:** The high concentration of antioxidants in black seed oil plays a pivotal role in protecting the skin from free radicals. This defense mechanism helps prevent oxidative stress, a key contributor to premature aging, and supports the skin's ability to maintain its youthful appearance.

- **Promotion of Collagen Production:** Black seed oil has been linked to the stimulation of collagen production. Collagen is essential for maintaining skin elasticity, and by promoting its synthesis, the oil contributes to reducing the appearance of fine lines and wrinkles.

4. Hyperpigmentation:

- **Evening Skin Tone:** Black seed oil's anti-inflammatory and antioxidant properties can contribute to a more even skin tone. By addressing inflammation and supporting overall skin health, it may aid in minimizing the appearance of hyperpigmentation.

5. Dry Skin:

- **Moisturizing Qualities:** Rich in omega-3 and omega-6 fatty acids, black seed oil is an effective natural moisturizer. It helps hydrate the skin, preventing dryness and flakiness, and promoting a smoother and more supple complexion.

6. Scarring:

- **Scar Reduction:** The regenerative properties of black seed oil may play a role in reducing the visibility of scars. Whether from acne or other skin injuries, consistent application of the oil may support the skin's natural healing processes.

Understanding the targeted benefits of black seed oil for common skin issues underscores its versatility as a natural remedy. Whether you're addressing acne, signs of aging, or skin conditions like eczema, the holistic properties of black seed oil offer a promising avenue for promoting skin health and radiance.

Incorporating Black Seed Oil into Your Skincare Routine: A Holistic Approach to Radiant Skin

1. *Choosing the Right Type of Black Seed Oil:*

- Opt for cold-pressed, organic black seed oil to ensure maximum retention of its beneficial compounds. Check for reputable brands with transparent sourcing practices to guarantee the purity and quality of the oil.

2. *Daily Cleansing:*

- Begin your skincare routine with a gentle cleanser to remove impurities. Add a few drops of black seed oil to your cleanser or apply it directly to damp skin. The oil's antimicrobial properties can assist in maintaining a clear complexion.

3. *Facial Serums:*

- Customize your own nourishing facial serum by combining black seed oil with other carrier oils like jojoba or rosehip. This blend can be applied morning and night, delivering a concentrated dose of antioxidants, fatty acids, and vitamins to support skin health.

4. *Masks and Treatments:*

- Create a rejuvenating face mask by mixing black seed oil with natural ingredients such as honey, yogurt, or aloe vera gel. Apply the mask weekly to promote hydration, soothe inflammation, and give your skin a radiant boost.

5. *Daily Moisturizers:*

- Enhance your daily moisturizer by adding a drop or two of black seed oil. This not only provides an extra layer of hydration but also infuses your skincare routine with the oil's nourishing and protective qualities.

6. *Spot Treatment for Blemishes:*

- For targeted care, apply a small amount of black seed oil directly to blemishes. The oil's antimicrobial and anti-inflammatory properties can aid in reducing redness and promoting the healing of acne spots.

7. *Under-eye Treatment:*

- Combat signs of fatigue and fine lines by gently tapping a drop of black seed oil around the eyes. Its moisturizing and collagen-boosting effects contribute to a brighter and more youthful under-eye area.

8. *Body Care:*

- Extend the benefits beyond your face by incorporating black seed oil into your body care routine. Add a few drops to your body lotion or apply the oil directly to damp skin after a shower for overall skin nourishment.

9. *Hair and Scalp Treatment:*

- Massage black seed oil into your scalp and hair to promote healthy hair growth and combat dryness. Its antimicrobial properties can also address dandruff and maintain a balanced scalp environment.

10. ***Internal Consumption:***

- Consider incorporating black seed oil into your diet for internal benefits. Whether consumed directly or added to smoothies and salads, internal use complements external application, offering a holistic approach to skin health.

11. ***Consistency is Key:***

- To reap the full rewards, consistency is paramount. Incorporate black seed oil into your skincare routine regularly, adjusting the concentration based on your skin's needs and sensitivities.

As you integrate black seed oil into your skincare ritual, embrace the opportunity to nurture your skin holistically. The adaptability of black seed oil allows for

a personalized approach, providing a versatile and
natural solution for a radiant and healthy complexion.

DIY Skincare Recipes and Applications with Black Seed Oil

1. *Nourishing Facial Serum:*

- *Ingredients:*

    - 1 tablespoon black seed oil

    - 1 tablespoon jojoba oil

    - 5 drops rosehip oil

    - 3 drops lavender essential oil

- *Instructions:*

    - Mix all the oils in a dark glass bottle.

    - Apply a few drops to your face and neck after cleansing, both in the morning and evening, for a nourishing and revitalizing serum.

2. *Hydrating Face Mask:*

- *Ingredients:*

  - 1 tablespoon black seed oil

  - 1 tablespoon honey

  - 1 tablespoon plain yogurt

- *Instructions:*

  - Combine the ingredients to form a smooth paste.

  - Apply the mask to your face, leave it on for 15-20 minutes, and then rinse with warm water. This mask helps hydrate and soothe the skin.

3. *Acne Spot Treatment:*

- *Ingredients:*

- 1 teaspoon black seed oil

- 1 drop tea tree essential oil

- *Instructions:*

  - Mix the oils and apply the blend directly to acne spots using a clean cotton swab.

  - Use this spot treatment in the evening before applying your moisturizer.

4. *Revitalizing Hair Mask:*

- *Ingredients:*

  - 2 tablespoons black seed oil

  - 1 tablespoon coconut oil

  - 1 egg

- *Instructions:*

  - Whisk the ingredients together and apply the mixture to your hair and scalp.

  - Leave the mask on for 30 minutes before washing your hair. This nourishing mask can help promote healthy hair and a balanced scalp.

5. Soothing Body Lotion:

- *Ingredients:*

  - 1/2 cup shea butter

  - 2 tablespoons black seed oil

  - 10 drops chamomile essential oil

- *Instructions:*

- Melt the shea butter, then let it cool slightly before adding the black seed oil and chamomile essential oil.

- Whip the mixture until it reaches a creamy consistency and store it in a jar. Use it as a soothing body lotion for dry or irritated skin.

6. *Under-eye Brightening Serum:*

- *Ingredients:*

  - 1 teaspoon black seed oil

  - 1 teaspoon sweet almond oil

  - 1 drop rose essential oil

- *Instructions:*

  - Combine the oils and apply a small amount gently around the eyes.

- Use this serum as part of your nighttime skincare routine for a hydrating and brightening effect.

7. *Lip Balm for Dry Lips:*

- *Ingredients:*

    - 1 tablespoon black seed oil

    - 1 tablespoon coconut oil

    - 1 tablespoon beeswax

- *Instructions:*

    - Melt the beeswax, then add the black seed oil and coconut oil.

    - Pour the mixture into small lip balm containers and let it solidify. Use this natural lip balm to keep your lips moisturized.

8. *Cleansing Oil for Makeup Removal:*

- *Ingredients:*

  - 1 tablespoon black seed oil

  - 1 tablespoon jojoba oil

- *Instructions:*

  - Mix the oils and use the blend to gently massage your face to remove makeup.

  - Rinse your face with warm water after massaging. This cleansing oil effectively removes makeup while leaving the skin nourished.

Experiment with these DIY recipes to discover the transformative potential of black seed oil in your skincare routine. Tailor the recipes to your preferences and skin needs, and enjoy the benefits of incorporating this natural elixir into your self-care rituals.

Potential Side Effects and Precautions When Using Black Seed Oil

While black seed oil is generally considered safe for topical and internal use, it's crucial to be aware of potential side effects and take necessary precautions to ensure a positive and safe experience. Here are some considerations:

1. Allergic Reactions:

- Individuals with known allergies to plants in the Ranunculaceae family, which includes black cumin (Nigella Sativa), should exercise caution. Allergic reactions may include skin rashes, itching, or respiratory issues. Perform a patch test before widespread use.

2. Gastrointestinal Upset:

- In some cases, oral consumption of black seed oil may lead to gastrointestinal discomfort such as nausea or stomach upset. Start with a small amount and gradually increase the dosage to assess your tolerance.

3. Blood Sugar Levels:

- People with diabetes should monitor their blood sugar levels closely when using black seed oil, as it may lower blood sugar. Consult with a healthcare professional before incorporating it into your routine, especially if you are taking medications for diabetes.

4. Blood Pressure:

- Black seed oil may have a mild hypotensive effect, potentially lowering blood pressure.

Black Seed Oil for Skin Treatment

Individuals with low blood pressure or those taking medication for hypertension should consult a healthcare provider before using black seed oil regularly.

5. Pregnancy and Breastfeeding:

- Pregnant or breastfeeding women should exercise caution and consult with a healthcare professional before using black seed oil. While there's some evidence suggesting potential benefits, safety during these periods has not been definitively established.

6. Surgery and Blood Clotting:

- Black seed oil might have mild antiplatelet effects. If you are scheduled for surgery or have a bleeding disorder, inform your healthcare provider about your use of black seed oil to prevent potential complications.

7. Interactions with Medications:

- Black seed oil may interact with certain medications, including anticoagulants, antiplatelet drugs, and hypoglycemic medications. Consult with a healthcare professional if you are taking any medications to avoid potential interactions.

8. Skin Sensitivity:

- While black seed oil is generally well-tolerated, individuals with sensitive skin may experience irritation. Perform a patch test before applying it to larger areas and dilute it with a carrier oil if necessary.

9. Quality and Purity:

- Ensure you are using high-quality, pure black seed oil. Choose reputable brands and check for certifications to guarantee that the oil is free from contaminants and additives.

10. Children:

- Use caution when considering black seed oil for children. Consult with a pediatrician before incorporating it into their skincare or dietary routines.

Before making black seed oil a regular part of your skincare or wellness routine, it's advisable to consult with a healthcare professional, especially if you have pre-existing health conditions or are taking medications. This proactive approach ensures that you can enjoy the potential benefits of black seed oil while

minimizing any potential risks or adverse effects.

Beyond Skin Deep: Exploring the Diverse Health Benefits of Black Seed Oil

Beyond its acclaimed role in skincare, black seed oil, derived from the seeds of Nigella Sativa, harbors a wealth of health benefits that extend far beyond the surface. As we delve into the broader spectrum of its applications, a multifaceted tapestry of well-being unfolds.

1. Immune System Support:

- Black seed oil has been recognized for its immune-modulating properties, helping to bolster the body's natural defense mechanisms. Its immune-enhancing effects are attributed to compounds like thymoquinone, making it a potential ally in fortifying resilience against various infections.

2. Cardiovascular Benefits:

- Research suggests that black seed oil may contribute to cardiovascular health by positively influencing lipid profiles. Its impact on cholesterol levels, blood pressure, and arterial function showcases its potential as a supportive element in maintaining a healthy heart.

3. Respiratory Health:

- The anti-inflammatory and antimicrobial properties of black seed oil make it a contender in promoting respiratory health. It may offer relief for conditions such as asthma, bronchitis, or allergies, helping to soothe airway inflammation and support easier breathing.

4. Digestive Aid:

- Traditionally used to alleviate digestive discomfort, black seed oil may aid in promoting a healthy digestive system. Its anti-inflammatory properties could contribute to soothing conditions like indigestion or bloating, fostering overall gastrointestinal well-being.

5. Anti-Inflammatory Effects:

- Systemic inflammation is implicated in various chronic conditions. Black seed oil's potent anti-inflammatory effects extend beyond the skin, potentially offering relief for inflammatory disorders such as arthritis and other autoimmune conditions.

6. Antioxidant Defense:

- The robust antioxidant profile of black seed oil plays a crucial role in neutralizing free radicals throughout the body. By mitigating oxidative stress, it contributes to cellular health and may reduce the risk of chronic diseases associated with oxidative damage.

7. Weight Management:

- Preliminary research suggests that black seed oil may aid in weight management by influencing factors such as appetite control, metabolism, and insulin sensitivity. However, more studies are needed to fully understand its impact on body weight.

8. Diabetes Support:

- Black seed oil has demonstrated potential in supporting individuals with diabetes by helping regulate blood sugar levels. Its hypoglycemic effects make it an area of interest for those seeking natural approaches to diabetes management.

9. Anti-Cancer Properties:

- While further research is needed, early studies suggest that black seed oil may exhibit anti-cancer properties. Thymoquinone, in particular, has shown promising effects in inhibiting the growth of certain cancer cells.

10. Joint Health:

- The anti-inflammatory and antioxidant properties of black seed oil may contribute to joint health. It has been explored for its potential in managing conditions like rheumatoid arthritis, providing relief from joint pain and stiffness.

As we unravel the diverse health benefits of black seed oil, it becomes evident that its impact extends to numerous facets of well-being. From immune support to cardiovascular health and beyond, black seed oil emerges as a holistic ally in nurturing a healthier and more resilient body. However, it's crucial to approach these potential benefits with a balanced perspective, recognizing that individual responses may vary, and more research is needed to fully elucidate the extent of black seed oil's therapeutic potential. Always consult with a healthcare professional before incorporating it into your wellness routine, especially if you have existing health conditions or are taking medications.

The Future of Black Seed Oil in Skincare: A Natural Renaissance

In the ever-evolving landscape of skincare, the future promises a continued and elevated role for black seed oil, heralding a natural renaissance in beauty and well-being. As we peer into the horizon, several trends and developments suggest an even more prominent place for this ancient elixir.

1. Sustainable and Ethical Formulations:

- The global shift towards sustainability and ethical sourcing is influencing skincare choices. Black seed oil, often sourced from organic and environmentally conscious producers, aligns seamlessly with this trend. As consumers increasingly seek products with transparent supply chains and minimal ecological impact, the ethical cultivation of black seed oil positions it as a frontrunner in conscientious skincare.

2. Advanced Formulations and Innovations:

- The integration of black seed oil into advanced skincare formulations is on the horizon. As research continues to unveil its intricate chemical composition and therapeutic potential, we can anticipate the development of innovative products that harness the synergistic benefits of black seed oil alongside cutting-edge skincare technologies.

3. Personalized Skincare:

- The future of skincare lies in personalization, acknowledging that individuals have unique skin types and concerns. Black seed oil's versatility makes it an ideal candidate for inclusion in personalized skincare routines, where formulations can be tailored to address specific needs, from acne-prone skin to anti-aging concerns.

4. Integration with Traditional and Modern Medicine:

- The convergence of traditional wisdom and modern scientific understanding will play a pivotal role in shaping the future of skincare. Black seed oil, deeply rooted in ancient healing traditions, is poised to be further embraced and validated through ongoing scientific research, establishing its credibility in both traditional and modern skincare practices.

5. Clinical Validation and Dermatological Endorsements:

- As black seed oil gains popularity, we can expect increased attention from the dermatological community. Clinical studies and dermatologist endorsements may pave the way for a more widespread acceptance of black seed oil as a valuable component in evidence-based skincare regimens.

6. Inclusion in Mainstream Beauty Brands:

- Mainstream beauty brands are likely to embrace the allure of black seed oil. With a growing demand for natural and holistic ingredients, beauty conglomerates may incorporate this versatile oil into their formulations, bringing its benefits to a wider audience.

7. DIY Skincare Culture:

- The DIY skincare movement, fueled by the desire for simplicity and self-expression, is expected to continue thriving. Black seed oil, with its adaptability and ease of incorporation into homemade remedies, will likely remain a staple in the DIY skincare culture.

8. Educational Resources and Consumer Awareness:

- The future holds an increased focus on consumer education and awareness. Resources elucidating the benefits of black seed oil, along with clear guidelines for usage, will empower individuals to make informed choices, fostering a deeper understanding of this ancient remedy.

As the future unfolds, black seed oil stands poised at the intersection of tradition and innovation, offering a bridge between the timeless wisdom of the past and the dynamic advancements of the present. Its journey through centuries attests to its enduring relevance, and the chapters yet to be written hold the promise of further discoveries, validations, and a continued legacy in the realm of skincare and holistic well-being.

Ongoing Research and Potential Developments in Black Seed Oil

As black seed oil gains recognition for its diverse therapeutic properties, ongoing research endeavors continue to unravel its intricacies and explore its potential applications. The evolving landscape of scientific inquiry hints at several areas of interest and potential developments.

1. Skin Microbiome Interaction:

- Research is delving into the interaction between black seed oil and the skin microbiome. Understanding how this natural elixir influences the delicate balance of microorganisms on the skin may provide insights into its mechanisms of action and potential for maintaining skin health.

2. Bioavailability Studies:

- Improving our understanding of the bioavailability of black seed oil's active compounds is a key focus. Research may explore optimal delivery methods and formulations to enhance the absorption of beneficial components, ensuring they reach target tissues and exert their therapeutic effects more effectively.

3. Comparative Studies with Conventional Treatments:

- Comparative studies between black seed oil and conventional skincare treatments are likely to expand. Investigating its efficacy in comparison to standard dermatological interventions may shed light on its role as a complementary or alternative option for various skin conditions.

4. Molecular Mechanisms in Anti-Aging:

- The molecular mechanisms underlying black seed oil's potential anti-aging effects are of particular interest. Unraveling how it influences collagen production, oxidative stress pathways, and cellular regeneration may pave the way for targeted anti-aging formulations.

5. Clinical Trials for Specific Skin Conditions:

- Conducting clinical trials focused on specific skin conditions, such as acne, eczema, or psoriasis, can provide more robust evidence regarding the effectiveness of black seed oil. Rigorous trials may explore optimal dosages, treatment durations, and potential side effects.

6. Exploration of Synergies with Other Natural Ingredients:

- Research may delve into synergistic effects when combining black seed oil with other natural ingredients. Combinations that enhance its efficacy or address a broader range of skin concerns may emerge, contributing to the development of advanced skincare formulations.

7. Genetic and Personalized Skincare Studies:

- Genetic studies exploring individual responses to black seed oil may become more prevalent. This personalized approach could lead to tailored skincare recommendations based on an individual's genetic makeup, optimizing outcomes and minimizing potential adverse effects.

8. Consumer Perception and Preferences:

- Research on consumer perception, preferences, and experiences with black seed oil in skincare will likely expand. Understanding how users incorporate it into their routines, their perceived benefits, and any challenges they encounter can guide product development and consumer education.

9. Exploration of Anti-Cancer Potential:

- The potential anti-cancer properties of black seed oil, as indicated by preliminary studies, may prompt further exploration. Ongoing research may focus on specific types of cancer, mechanisms of action, and the development of adjunctive therapies.

10. Impact on Mental Health and Well-Being:

- Beyond physical health, emerging research may explore the impact of black seed oil on mental health and well-being. Investigations into its potential neuroprotective and mood-regulating effects could broaden its applications to holistic self-care.

As these research trajectories unfold, the future holds the promise of a more comprehensive understanding of black seed oil's potential in skincare and overall well-being. From molecular insights to clinical applications, ongoing studies are likely to shape its role in diverse therapeutic landscapes, offering a tapestry of possibilities for the natural elixir derived from Nigella

Sativa.

Emerging Trends in Natural Skincare: Nurturing Beauty Holistically

As consumers increasingly gravitate toward clean, sustainable, and holistic beauty practices, the world of natural skincare is witnessing a transformative shift. Emerging trends reflect a profound connection between nature, science, and self-care, signaling a new era in the way we approach skincare.

1. Biophilic Beauty:

- *Concept:* Inspired by biophilia, the innate human connection with nature, biophilic beauty emphasizes formulations that mimic the natural environment. Expect products with botanical textures, earthy scents, and eco-friendly packaging.

2. Upcycled Beauty:

- *Concept:* Upcycled beauty focuses on repurposing waste by-products from the food and cosmetic industries. Brands are exploring innovative ways to use discarded materials to create sustainable and effective skincare products.

3. Blue Beauty and Marine Ingredients:

- *Concept:* Blue beauty aligns with ocean conservation, promoting marine-friendly ingredients and sustainable sourcing. Expect skincare formulations featuring seaweed, algae, and other marine extracts known for their nourishing and rejuvenating properties.

4. Cannabinoid Skincare:

- *Concept:* Cannabinoids, derived from hemp and cannabis plants, are gaining popularity for their potential anti-inflammatory and soothing effects. Cannabinoid-infused skincare products are emerging as a trend, aiming to provide holistic relief and balance.

5. Skin Microbiome-Friendly Products:

- *Concept:* With a growing understanding of the skin microbiome's role in skin health, skincare formulations are shifting towards products that support and maintain a healthy balance of skin microorganisms.

6. Adaptogens in Skincare:

- *Concept:* Adaptogens, known for their stress-regulating properties, are finding their way into skincare. Ingredients like ashwagandha and rhodiola are being incorporated to address the impact of stress on skin health.

7. DIY and Customization:

- *Concept:* The DIY skincare trend continues to flourish, emphasizing self-expression and personalization. Brands are offering customization options, allowing consumers to tailor products to their unique skin needs and preferences.

8. Waterless Beauty:

- *Concept:* Water scarcity concerns have led to the rise of waterless beauty products. Formulations are becoming more concentrated, utilizing potent botanical extracts and oils, reducing the need for water as a primary ingredient.

9. Indigenous Ingredients and Rituals:

- *Concept:* Brands are exploring the wealth of traditional knowledge and indigenous ingredients. Skincare formulations inspired by ancient rituals and locally sourced ingredients are gaining popularity for their cultural significance and unique benefits.

10. Tech-Enhanced Natural Skincare:

- *Concept:* The fusion of technology and nature is giving rise to tech-enhanced natural skincare. From AI-powered skin analysis for personalized recommendations to smart devices optimizing product application, technology is becoming an integral part of the natural skincare experience.

11. Regenerative Agriculture and Soil Health:

- *Concept:* Regenerative agriculture practices, which prioritize soil health and biodiversity, are influencing ingredient sourcing. Brands committed to sustainability are choosing suppliers who embrace regenerative farming methods.

12. Holistic Wellness Integration:

- *Concept:* Natural skincare is becoming a holistic wellness practice. Brands are recognizing the interconnectedness of physical and mental well-being, offering products that address both the external and internal aspects of beauty.

These emerging trends in natural skincare reflect a broader cultural shift towards mindful, sustainable, and personalized beauty practices. The intersection of nature, science, and well-being is reshaping the skincare landscape, offering a diverse array of options for those seeking a holistic and conscientious approach to self-care.

Conclusion

As we draw the final curtain on our exploration into the profound realm of black seed oil and its transformative impact on skincare and well-being, we find ourselves at the crossroads of tradition and modernity, ancient wisdom and contemporary science. The journey through these pages has been a voyage into the heart of natural healing, where the simplicity of an age-old remedy meets the complexity of our ever-evolving understanding of beauty and health.

In the chapters preceding this conclusion, we've traced the roots of black seed oil, delving into its historical significance and cultural tapestry. We've unraveled the intricate science behind its efficacy, understanding how its chemical composition harmonizes with the body's natural processes. From the intimate details of its role in addressing common skin issues to its broader impact on immune function, cardiovascular health, and beyond, black seed oil emerges not just as a skincare ally but as a holistic elixir for the body, mind, and spirit.

The resurgence of black seed oil in the contemporary skincare landscape is not merely a trend; it's a testament to the enduring power of nature's gifts. We've witnessed its revival from ancient traditions to the forefront of modern self-care rituals, driven by a collective yearning for authenticity and simplicity in our beauty routines.

Looking to the future, we see the potential for black seed oil to continue its ascent, not just as a fleeting trend but as a timeless pillar in the realm of natural wellness. The ongoing research and evolving trends in skincare affirm its relevance, promising new insights and applications that will further elevate its standing in the beauty and wellness spheres.

As we bid farewell to these pages, let us carry with us the profound understanding that beauty is not a mere surface-level pursuit but a holistic journey that embraces the essence of tradition, the wisdom of nature, and the advancements of science. Whether you embark on this journey with a drop of black seed oil on your skin or with the intention to nurture your well-being from within, may it be a voyage filled with self-discovery, self-care, and the radiant glow that comes from embracing the timeless harmony between humanity and the natural world.